The Simplest Low Carb Recipe Book

Healthy and Delicious Recipes with Easy-Follow 14-Day Meal Plan

Emily Pride

Table of Contents

EXCLUSIVE BONUS

40 Weight Loss Recipes

&

14 Days Meal Plan

Scan the QR-Code and receive
the FREE download:

Introduction

If you don't yet know much about low carbs and how a low carb lifestyle works, we are going to dip into this before plunging into the recipes. It's really important to note before starting that while you may be able to increase your health by reducing how many carbs you eat, low carb does not mean no carb. You need carbohydrates to survive and function, and you must not try to get rid of all the carbs from your diet – you will get very ill. Low carb eating has many advantages, but it should not be taken to the extremes. Like all diets, moderation is key to safety.

Before you consider starting on a low carb diet, you should discuss the diet and its realities with your doctor and ask for advice. This is particularly true if you have any health conditions like diabetes, but it stands for anyone. Radically altering how many carbs you consume will have a lot of implications for your health and while it may offer benefits, you should talk to a doctor before you do anything else. It is always a good idea to discuss dramatic changes to your diet with your doctor to see what health implications there may be. You should follow this up with further discussions once you have begun the diet.

What Is A Low Carb Lifestyle?

There are quite a few different kinds of lifestyles that count as low carb. Many people have different interpretations of this term, and what counts as "low carb" can be quite varied. A lot of it depends on your perspective and the kind of foods you are used to. If you eat a lot of foods that are high in carbohydrates, you might find it helps to start with a medium carb diet to begin with, and work toward low carb – or at least to choose meals that are at the higher end of the low carb diet.

Some low carb diets suggest eating fewer than 130 g of carbohydrates every day. A large jacket potato could contain as many as 90 g of carbs, while an apple only contains around 20 g. Choosing what foods you eat will be even more important than moderating the quantities. Some foods are likely to disappear from your menu entirely, while others may just be much more limited.

Remember that it is okay to eat a meal that is higher in carbs as long as you pair this with other low carb options throughout the day. If you are craving particular foods, cut back your carbs in other meals so that you can enjoy at least some of them from time to time – this is a great way to make your diet more flexible and more sustainable.

What Types Of Low Carb Lifestyles Are There?

There are lots of different kinds of low carb diets out there, and which you follow will depend on what suits you best. Below are a few of the options:

1) Standard low carb diet:

This diet does not have a fixed definition, but in general, it suggests eating between 50 g and 150 g of carbohydrates each day. 100-150 g is considered a good amount for maintaining your current weight, while 50-100 g will aid slow weight loss, and under 50 g is intended to encourage fast weight loss. Which of these options you choose will depend on your situation and preferences, but be cautious if you are choosing the 50 g option.

2) Low carb, high fat:

Often known as LCHF, this diet is about keeping your carbs very low and eating a lot of unprocessed, whole foods, such as eggs, vegetables, meat, berries, and shellfish. Many people following this diet will eat as few as 20 carbs per day (although it may go up to 100) and often consume a lot of fat instead.

3) Ketogenic diet:

You have almost certainly heard of the ketogenic diet, which is also low carb, high fat. It is aimed at decreasing your insulin levels and getting your body to run on ketones, which are made by the body releasing fat from its stores to produce energy. This diet is thought to have some benefits for certain kinds of epilepsy, but it has also become popular among dieters and bodybuilders because it is a good way to lose weight fast. It often involves eating fewer than 50 carbs per day, and may be as low as 20 or 30.

4) Atkins diet:

This is the most commonly recognized low carb diet, and it restricts carbs but not protein or fat. It has four phases, including the induction phase, where you eat fewer than 20 carbs per day for 2 weeks; the balancing phase, where you gradually add more fruits, nuts, and low carb vegetables; the fine-tuning phase, where you add a few more carbs back in to curb your weight loss; and the maintenance phase, where you eat as many carbs as you need to sustain the weight loss you have achieved.

5) Eco-Atkins diet:

If you are vegan, there is a version of the Atkins diet that is suitable for you as well. This is actually thought to be healthier than the Atkins diet, although it is higher in carbs overall. It incorporates a lot of plant proteins, such as soya, and plant oils.

6) Low carb paleo diet:

Following a paleo diet has become very popular in recent years, and this diet involves eating foods that our ancestors would have eaten. The theory is that we are not adapted to modern foods yet, and we can stay healthier by choosing foods that we originally evolved to eat, such as unprocessed vegetables, tubers, nuts, and seeds. Meat and fish are also fine, as are eggs. Processed foods, such as dairy, legumes, and added sugar are not eaten.

The paleo diet in itself is not low carb, but by selecting the right vegetables, it is easy to adapt, and many people choose to do this.

7) Low carb Mediterranean diet:

The Mediterranean diet has been given a lot of attention by health professionals, and it is thought to have some ability to reduce your risk of heart disease, type 2 diabetes, and breast cancer. This diet is popular, but the low carb version is a little more complicated because it involves cutting out grains and choosing fatty fish instead of red meat. It is not particularly different to the standard low carb diet, but it tends to include more fish and plant oils.

8) Zero carb diet:

This is one of the most extreme carbohydrate-focused diets, and it involves completely removing carbs from your diet. However, there is not currently much evidence to show that this is safe, let alone healthy, and a zero carb diet involves eating exclusively animal-based foods. You will not eat any plants if you follow a zero carb diet, and this can lead to major deficiencies in vitamins and other nutrients. This diet is not recommended for anyone.

What Products Are Allowed When Following A Low Carb Lifestyle?

Having a rough idea of what you can and can't eat on a low carb diet is useful. This diet is popular, but one of the frustrating things about it is that it is rarely defined thoroughly enough for people to follow it strictly, and that can leave some people feeling out of control and uncertain about their meals. You may find it helps to have lists of certain foods that are definitely okay (provided you are eating them in the right quantities). Here are some "approved" low carb foods for you to try:

- Unsweetened dairy products (e.g. Greek yoghurt / yogurt, whole milk)
- Cauliflower
- Broccoli
- Lean meats (e.g. chicken breasts, pork)
- Fish

- Eggs
- Nuts and seeds
- Nut butters
- Oils
- Leafy greens
- Fruits
- Vegetables that grow above ground

If you use these products as the foundations of your diet, you should have plenty of options to choose between, which should make following the diet easier.

What about foods that you can't eat? It may also be useful to have some ideas about the foods you should try to avoid. Note that it's still okay to sometimes have these foods in small quantities and being a little flexible can sometimes make it easier to stick to a diet, but on the whole, you should try to avoid foods in the following groups:

- Pasta
- Bread
- Rice
- Oats
- Cereal
- Potatoes
- Beans
- Carrots

- Sugary drinks
- Sugary dairy products
- Low-fat products (these tend to be high in sugar)

What Are The Advantages Of A Low Carb Lifestyle?

You might be wondering what you actually stand to gain by following a low carb lifestyle, and the answer is that there are a variety of advantages that tend to be associated with this kind of eating. Let's explore some of them.

1) Improved weight loss:

Low carb diets are often used as a means of helping individuals to lose weight. Several studies have now shown that a low carb diet can help you lose weight more quickly and effectively than a low fat diet, although this tends to be most noticeable when you begin the diet, rather than later on. This is because it has a quick impact, lowering your insulin levels and getting rid of excess water in the body. In the long term, a low carb diet isn't noticeably more effective than other diets, but for short term weight loss, it's superior.

2) Increased HDL cholesterol:

You probably already know that HDL is the "good" kind of cholesterol, because it helps to lower your LDL (the "bad" cholesterol), and this reduces your risk of heart disease. Fatty foods are a good way to increase HDL, and low carb diets tend to include lots of fat.

3) Reduced LDL cholesterol:

Having read the above, it won't surprise you to learn that a low carb diet can help you reduce your LDL levels, but there's a little more to it than this. It has been shown that small particles of LDL are more dangerous and potentially damaging than large ones, and a low carb diet will both reduce the overall number of LDL particles and increase the size of those that remain in your bloodstream. This will improve your overall health.

4) Reduced risk of metabolic syndrome:

Metabolic syndrome is frequently associated with the risk of heart disease and diabetes, and a low carb diet is effective at reducing your risk of developing this condition. Metabolic syndrome can cause a variety of issues, including low HDL levels, elevated blood sugar levels while fasting, and abdominal obesity – so a low carb diet could be useful if you are struggling with these symptoms.

5) Lower triglycerides:

You may be familiar with the term triglycerides. These are molecules of fat found in the bloodstream, and if the levels in your blood remain high even when you fast overnight, you are at a far greater risk of heart disease. Reducing the number of carbs you eat can quickly and dramatically reduce the number of triglycerides in your blood. Getting rid of fructose from your diet is a particularly good way to lower the triglycerides.

6) Reduced appetite:

Often, diets leave people feeling hungry and unsatisfied after a meal, because you are changing what you eat and usually reducing the quantities. This makes it hard to sustain a diet, and causes a lot of people to give up after a relatively short amount of time.

However, this doesn't occur with a low carb diet, because this kind of diet automatically curbs your appetite. Protein and fat will make you feel fuller faster, while you need a lot of carbohydrates to feel full. By swapping carbs for protein, you will find that you need less food, and don't get hungry as quickly. This makes a low carb diet noticeably more sustainable than many other diet options.

7) Loss of abdominal weight:

Abdominal fat is one of the biggest issues that people face, and it can cause a lot of health problems. The fat that collects around the abdomen is known as visceral fat, and this tends to lodge around organs and cause metabolic dysfunction. It is more important to try to reduce this kind of fat than other kinds of fat (subcutaneous fat), and a low carb diet is one of the most efficient ways to do this.

8) Reduction in blood sugar levels:

Many people suffer from insulin resistance and diabetes, and a low carb diet can help with this too. It reduces the blood sugar levels dramatically, which could lower your risk of diabetes, or help you to manage it if you already suffer from this condition.

Remember to talk to a doctor if you have a condition that means you need to monitor your blood sugar levels, as a low carb diet could cause unpredictable spikes or drops.

9) Reduction in insulin:

Like the reduction in blood sugar levels, this can be of value to people who suffer from high insulin levels. Reducing your carbohydrate intake will lower the levels of insulin in your blood very quickly. Again, discuss this with a doctor if you have any health conditions.

10) Lowering blood pressure:

High blood pressure can be a major issue that puts you at risk of many different health conditions, including kidney failure, hypertension, strokes, and heart disease. Reducing how many carbs you eat will help to bring your blood pressure down, making you healthier.

As you can see, there are many advantages to swapping to a low carb diet, and it can help with a whole host of health conditions, as well as reducing your risk of developing these conditions in the first place. However, a low carb diet can be challenging to achieve, so we're going to find some healthy recipes that will get you started and give you a foundation to work from as you begin making changes to your eating routines.

TASTY LOW CARB BREAKFAST IDEAS

Breakfast might be the most important meal of the day, but it's one that many people find difficult. Breakfast is often rushed, marred by the grogginess of early mornings, enforced wake-ups, and the chaos of getting everything you need for the day ready so you can step out of the door on time. However, setting yourself up to succeed all day means taking the time to get a good breakfast. It doesn't have to be complicated, but if you're used to jamming a slice of bread in the toaster or throwing together some cereal, you will need to rethink things a bit.

With that in mind, let's find some simple, easy breakfast meals you can try. It doesn't have to be complicated to be filling and tasty.

Cream Cheese Pancakes

You can't eat ordinary pancakes with flour, but you can enjoy these simple, fluffy pancakes made with cream cheese, and they only take a little while to whip up.

Serves: 1

You will need:

- 1 teaspoon of vanilla extract
- 2 eggs
- 2 tablespoons of olive oil
- 60 g / 2 oz of cream cheese
- ½ teaspoon of sugar

Method:

1 Get out your food processor and add all of the ingredients, except the olive oil. If you don't have a food processor, you can beat the mixture by hand in a large mixing bowl.

2 When the mixture is smooth, heat the oil in a large skillet over a medium heat and pour ¼ of the batter in once the oil is hot.

3 Cook for about 3 minutes on one side and then flip the pancake and cook for another 2-3 minutes. Remove the pancake from the pan and add another ¼ of the batter.

4 Continue until you have four pancakes and then top with your favourite options.

Nutritional info:

Calories: 600

Fat: 57.5 g

Cholesterol: 434 mg

Sodium: 308 mg

Carbohydrates: 4.8 g

Fibre: 0 g

Protein: 16.9 g

Banana Bread

You won't be eating traditional banana bread for breakfast, but it's possible to make a low carb version of this snack, and this makes for a super easy breakfast on any day of the week. You can also slice and freeze it, and then toast it to enjoy it hot and crispy – or take a few slices cold to work with you. It's very versatile and a great low carb option for the days when you don't want to cook.

> Serves: 6

You will need:

- 50 g / ½ cup of almond flour
- 3 bananas
- 3 eggs
- 120 g / ½ cup of almond butter
- 1 tablespoon of cinnamon
- 1 teaspoon of vanilla extract
- 1 teaspoon of baking soda
- 1 teaspoon of baking powder
- 4 tablespoons of melted butter

Method:

1. Preheat your oven to 230 degrees C / 450 degrees F.

2. Mash your bananas thoroughly into a smooth mush.

3. Mix the almond butter into the bananas.

4. Melt your butter in a microwave or over the stove and mix this in too.

5. Crack the eggs into the bowl and mix well, and then add the vanilla extract.

6. Add the almond flour, baking powder, baking soda, and cinnamon to the bowl and stir thoroughly.

7. Grease a loaf tin and pour the batter in, and then bake for 45 minutes.

8. Insert a toothpick to check that it comes out clean, and then take the banana bread out of the oven and place it on the counter to cool for 10 minutes. Turn it out onto a cooling rack to finish cooling, and store in an airtight container.

Nutritional info (based on slicing loaf into 6 slices):

Calories: 222

Fat: 15.2 g

Cholesterol: 102 mg

Sodium: 398 mg

Carbohydrates: 17.3 g

Fibre: 3.3 g

Protein: 5.8 g

Baked Egg Avocados

If you love avocados, these bacon and egg filled avocado halves make a great start to the day, and they cook pretty quickly, so they should work even if you need to get out of the door promptly. You can alter the toppings a bit if you like, or make them vegetarian by leaving out the bacon – either way, they will be delicious.

Serves: 4

You will need:

- 4 eggs
- 2 avocados
- 55 g / ¼ cup of bacon
- 20 g / 4 teaspoons of cheddar cheese
- 1 tomato
- 1 teaspoon of basil
- Pinch of salt
- Pinch of pepper
- 2 tablespoons of chives

Method:

1 Preheat your oven to 200 degrees C / 400 degrees F.

2 Cut your avocados in half lengthwise and scoop out the pits. Leave the skins on.

3 Get out a baking sheet and place the avocado halves on it, facing up.

4 Use a spoon to enlarge the hole left by the pit. You can use this flesh up in other recipes if you choose.

5 Crack an egg into each avocado hole and season it, and then top it with bacon, slices of tomato, and a little cheddar cheese.

6 Place in the oven and bake for 15 minutes, or until egg yolks are cooked.

7 Chop your herbs and sprinkle them across the avocados to serve.

Nutritional info:

Calories: 369

Fat: 31.4 g

Cholesterol: 184 mg

Sodium: 457 mg

Carbohydrates: 10.5 g

Fibre: 7.2 g

Protein: 14.1 g

Toasted Nuts And Cottage Cheese Bowl

If you want a really simple throw-together breakfast, you might enjoy this fruity, nutty concoction that you can toss together in just a few minutes, especially if you toast the nuts in advance. If you would rather not toast the nuts, just skip that step. This is a little heavier on the carbs than some of the other breakfasts, but it makes a lovely change and is a very refreshing way to start the day.

Serves: 1

You will need:

- 110 g / ½ cup of low fat cottage cheese
- 90 g / ½ cup of 4% fat Greek yoghurt / yogurt
- 30 g / 1 oz of blueberries
- ½ teaspoon of vanilla extract
- 30 g / 1 oz of strawberries
- Pinch of cinnamon
- 15 g / ½ oz of almonds
- 15 g / ½ oz of walnuts

Method:

1 Toast your nuts in a dry, non-stick skillet over a medium heat. It should only take a few minutes. You can chop them first or leave them whole, and add spices like nutmeg if you want to make the dish more flavourful.

2 Add your cottage cheese and yoghurt / yogurt to a bowl.

3 Wash the blueberries and strawberries. Top, tail, and slice the strawberries, and stir them into the bowl, along with the blueberries.

4 Add the nuts and the pinch of cinnamon, plus a dash of vanilla extract, and enjoy.

Nutritional info:

Calories: 409
Fat: 20.6 g
Cholesterol: 16 mg
Sodium: 506 mg
Carbohydrates: 21 g
Fibre: 4.1 g
Protein: 36.5 g

Scrambled Eggs And Smoked Salmon

For a quick, easy, and satisfying breakfast, try some scrambled eggs and smoked salmon, but make sure you forgo the toast so you don't bump up the carbs. If necessary, add a few vegetables to make yourself feel fuller, like peas or green beans.

> Serves: 1

You will need:

- 2 eggs
- 50 g / 2 oz of smoked salmon
- Pinch of dill
- ½ tablespoon of butter
- Pinch of salt

Method:

1 Melt the butter in a small skillet above a medium heat. Tear up the smoked salmon and toss it into the pan to warm.

2 Crack your eggs into a cup and whisk them thoroughly until they are frothy and airy.

3 Pour the eggs into the pan and stir, constantly scraping the mixture into the centre of the pan and moving it around so that it cooks evenly and the salmon mixes through it.

4 Serve topped with dill and a touch of salt.

Nutritional info:

Calories: 243

Fat: 17 g

Cholesterol: 356 mg

Sodium: 1453 mg

Carbohydrates: 0.8 g

Fibre: 0 g

Protein: 21.5 g

Shakshuka

If you've never had shakshuka, you are in for a treat – this amazing recipe can be eaten at any time of the day, but it's a particularly popular breakfast recipe. You can have it hot or cold, so feel free to make it for dinner and then enjoy the leftovers for breakfast the following day, or make it for a lazy weekend breakfast. It's a truly delicious option that's naturally low in carbs.

Serves: 6

You will need:

- 1 medium onion
- 2 tablespoons of olive oil
- 1 red pepper
- 2 teaspoons of paprika
- 4 cloves of garlic
- 6 eggs
- 1 teaspoon of cumin
- 800 g / 28 oz whole peeled tinned tomatoes
- ¼ teaspoon of chilli powder
- 10 g fresh parsley
- 10 g fresh coriander / cilantro
- Pinch of salt
- Pinch of pepper

Method:

1 Wash your pepper and chop it. Peel and chop the onion.

2 Heat the olive oil in a large pan and fry the pepper and onion until the onion is turning translucent.

3 Peel and mince your garlic and add it to the pan, along with the spices. Fry for 2 minutes.

4 Add the tinned tomatoes into the pan and use a wooden spoon to break them up. Bring the sauce to a simmer for 5 minutes.

5 Use the spoon to make 6 wells around the pan, gently pushing the sauce to one side. Crack an egg into each well.

6 Cover the pan and cook for 5 minutes, and then check the eggs. They may need longer to be cooked to your liking.

7 Serve with a garnish of coriander / cilantro and parsley.

Nutritional info:
Calories: 159
Fat: 9.6 g
Cholesterol: 164 mg
Sodium: 389 mg
Carbohydrates: 13.2 g
Fibre: 2.5 g
Protein: 7.5 g

EXCLUSIVE BONUS

40 Weight Loss Recipes

&

14 Days Meal Plan

Scan the QR-Code and receive
the FREE download:

DELICIOUS LOW CARB LUNCHES

It's also important to keep your diet going when the middle of the day rolls around and you start to get peckish. At this point, it becomes all too easy to reach for a sandwich or a bag of carb-heavy crisps / chips – but you need to resist. Fortunately, there are plenty of great lunches you can try out instead.

Cheesy Mushrooms

If you want to make lunch quick and easy and you're looking to cut down on your meat, these cheesy baked mushrooms are ideal. Feel free to adapt the recipe if you want to add other vegetables in, but otherwise, this is ultra fast to make.

Serves: 4

You will need:

- 4 large mushrooms
- 25 g / 0.8 oz of walnuts
- 50 g rocket / 1 ½ oz arugula
- ½ teaspoon of thyme
- 100 g / 3 ½ oz of Gorgonzola or another blue cheese
- 10 g / 1/3 oz of butter
- 2 tomatoes

Method:

1. Preheat your oven to 200 degrees C / 400 degrees F.

2. Wash your mushrooms and shake them dry, and then place them on a baking tray, with the gills facing up.

3. In a dry skillet, lightly toast your walnuts for a few minutes. Chop into rough chunks once toasted.

4. Grate or crumble your Gorgonzola across the mushrooms, and then add the walnuts and thyme, plus a little butter.

5. Bake the mushrooms in the oven for 10 minutes and then serve with fresh, washed rocket / arugula.

Nutritional info:

Calories: 162

Fat: 13 g

Cholesterol: 29 mg

Sodium: 335 mg

Carbohydrates: 5.9 g

Fibre: 2.4 g

Protein: 8.6 g

Chicken Caesar Salad

Chicken Caesar salad makes a tasty lunch that is easy to transport if necessary, and it packs a great protein punch. It doesn't need heating, refreshing, or otherwise adding to once it is made, so you can put a few batches in the fridge and have some easy lunches ready to grab on any day of the week.

> Serves: 4

You will need:

- 2 tablespoons of olive oil
- 25 g / 0.8 oz of Parmesan
- 4 chicken breasts
- 4 eggs
- 1 Romaine lettuce
- 3 tablespoons of lemon juice
- 170 g / 6 oz of fat free Greek yoghurt / yogurt
- 50 g / 1 ½ oz of anchovy fillets
- 50 g / 1 ½ oz of watercress

Method:

1 Toss the chicken breasts with olive oil and a tablespoon of lemon juice, and allow them to rest for a couple of minutes. Season if you choose to.

2 Place the chicken breasts on a foil-lined tray and grill under a high heat for about 5 minutes. Turn the chicken breasts over and grill for another 5-6 minutes, until fully cooked (with an internal temperature of 74 degrees C / 165 degrees F).

3 Place on a board and allow to cool slightly, and then slice into strips or chunks.

4 Wash your lettuce and cress and set them aside to dry.

5 Boil 4 eggs until fully cooked and then cool, peel, and rinse. Cut into quarters.

6 Chop half of the anchovies and grate the Parmesan, and then mix these together with yoghurt / yogurt and lemon juice. Taste and alter the quantities if necessary.

7 Add the chicken breasts, lettuce, cress, egg quarters, and the yoghurt / yogurt mixture to a bowl, and top the salad with the remaining whole anchovies and enjoy.

Nutritional info:

Calories: 461
Fat: 20.8 g
Cholesterol: 309 mg
Sodium: 725 mg
Carbohydrates: 8 g
Fibre: 0.2 g
Protein: 59 g

Courgette / Zucchini Ragu With Poached Eggs

If you're fancying something packed with vegetables and you're at home to cook a hot lunch, this light ragu is perfect. You can use it as a side dish or spice it up with a little smoked meat if you like, but it's wonderfully light and simple in its basic form.

Serves: 6

You will need:

- 2 courgettes / zucchinis
- 3 cloves of garlic
- Pinch of salt
- Pinch of pepper
- 200 g / 7 oz of tomatoes
- 1 onion
- 115 g / 4 oz of mozzarella
- ¼ cup of basil leaves
- ¼ cup of parsley
- 6 tablespoons of olive oil
- 6 eggs

Method:

1 Place a large non-stick skillet over a medium heat and add the olive oil. Peel and chop your onion, and peel and mince the garlic.

2 When the oil starts to shimmer, add the onion and garlic and cook until soft and fragrant (about 8 minutes).

3 Wash and slice the courgettes / zucchinis and season them, and then toss them into the pan and gently fry until they turn golden.

4 Wash and chop your tomatoes and stir them into the pan. Cook until just soft, and check that the courgette / zucchini is also starting to soften.

5 Put on a second pan and bring a small quantity of water to the boil, and then crack your eggs into it. Poach lightly for a few minutes.

6 Roughly chop the mozzarella into chunks, and shred the basil and parsley.

7 Serve the sauce, topped with mozzarella chunks and herbs, and add the eggs on top.

Nutritional info:

Calories: 225

Fat: 19.6 g

Cholesterol: 167 mg

Sodium: 132 mg

Carbohydrates: 6.4 g

Fibre: 1.7 g

Protein: 8.6 g

Aubergine / Eggplant Pizza

Pizza is such a classic lunchtime recipe, but you can't eat it if you're following a low carb diet – so how else can you enjoy this delicious and easy meal? There are a few options, but if you really just want an excuse to pile up your favourite toppings and have some melted cheese, you're in luck, because aubergine / eggplant pizza is a great alternative.

Serves: 6

You will need:

- 1 aubergine / eggplant
- 80 ml / 1/3 cup of olive oil
- 280 g / 1 ¼ cups of marinara sauce
- ½ a red pepper
- 400 g / 2 cups of tomatoes
- 115 g / 4 oz of mozzarella
- 3 teaspoons of fresh basil
- Pinch of salt
- Pinch of pepper

Method:

1. Preheat your oven to 200 degrees C / 400 degrees F.

2. Wash your aubergine / eggplant and remove the ends, and then slice into ¾ inch rounds. Place the slices on a tray and brush both sides generously with olive oil, and then season.

3. Place them in the oven and roast for about 11 minutes until they start to become tender.

4. Wash and halve your tomatoes and wash and slice the red pepper.

5. Take the aubergine / eggplant out of the oven and top it with marinara sauce.

6. Add the tomatoes and red pepper, and then sprinkle grated mozzarella across the top.

7. Roast for another 6 minutes, until the cheese is melting and the tomatoes and peppers are cooked.

8. Serve hot with a sprinkling of basil and extra salt or pepper if you like.

Nutritional info:

Calories: 207
Fat: 14.4 g
Cholesterol: 5 mg
Sodium: 331 mg
Carbohydrates: 17.3 g
Fibre: 5.7 g
Protein: 4.7 g

Mediterranean Mackerel Salad

If you want to get some oily fish into your lunches, mackerel is a great option, and this salad is perfect for making in advance and keeping in the fridge. You can alter the ingredients if there are any you don't like, or try an addition of chopped olives or sun-dried tomatoes to spice it up a bit.

Serves: 6

You will need:

- 2 tins of mackerel in sunflower oil
- ½ red onion
- 1/3 cup of parsley
- 2 teaspoons of capers
- 30 g / ¼ cup of feta cheese
- 1 cucumber
- ½ avocado
- 410 g / 14 ½ oz of tinned chickpeas (drain and rinse)
- ¼ teaspoon of black pepper
- Pinch of salt
- 150 g / 1 cup of roasted red peppers

To make the vinaigrette, you will need:

- 2 tablespoons of red wine vinegar
- 2 tablespoons of olive oil
- 1 teaspoon of oregano
- 1 teaspoon of parsley
- 1 teaspoon of lemon juice
- ¼ teaspoon of black pepper
- Pinch of salt

Method:

1   Drain your mackerel and tip it into a large bowl.

2   Wash and chop your cucumber, red peppers, parsley, red onion, and avocado, and crumble the feta cheese.

3   Add all of the ingredients to the mackerel's bowl and stir to combine.

4   To make the vinaigrette, in a separate bowl, whisk together chopped parsley and oregano, lemon juice, black pepper, salt, olive oil, and red wine vinegar. Taste and adjust if necessary, and then drizzle generously across your salad.

Nutritional info:

Calories: 291

Fat: 17 g

Cholesterol. 6 mg

Sodium: 650 mg

Carbohydrates: 24.2 g

Fibre: 5.7 g

Protein: 12.6 g

EXCELLENT LOW CARB DINNER RECIPES

For many people, dinner is the treat at the end of the day, and if that's the case for you, you may not feel like sticking to your diet. It's all too easy to slip up and undo your hard work with all the tempting high carb foods that we often eat for dinner. Things like pasta, pizza, baked potatoes, and rice dishes are convenient foods, but they aren't ideal for this diet – so let's find some other great recipes for you to enjoy.

Garlic-Infused Shrimp And Broccoli

If you're looking for a one-pot meal to impress, this garlic, shrimp, and broccoli meal is perfect, and it should only take about 20 minutes to hit the table, so it will work well if you're rushing in the evening. Make sure you're using nice, fresh broccoli for maximum flavour!

Serves: 4

You will need:

- 3 teaspoons of lemon juice
- 6 cloves of garlic
- 3 tablespoons of extra-virgin olive oil
- 365 g / 4 cups of broccoli florets
- 75 g / ½ cup of red pepper
- 450 g / 1 lb of shrimps (peeled, deveined)
- ½ teaspoon of black pepper
- ½ teaspoon of salt

Method:

1. Add 2 tablespoons of olive oil to a pan and warm it over a medium heat. Peel and mince your garlic and add half of it to the pan, and cook for 1 minute.

2. Wash and chop your broccoli and peppers and add them to the pan, with half of the salt and half of the pepper.

3. Cover the pan and cook for about 5 minutes until the vegetables are soft. If necessary, add a splash of water to prevent them from sticking or burning.

4. When cooked, tip them into a bowl and cover to keep them warm.

5. Turn up the heat a little and add the rest of the oil to the pan. Toss in the rest of the garlic and cook for 1 minute, and then add the shrimps and the rest of the salt and pepper.

6. Stir and cook for about 5 minutes, making sure the shrimps get flipped and cooked on both sides. When the shrimps are cooked, add the broccoli mixture back to the pan and mix everything together. Add the lemon juice and heat it all up, and then serve.

Nutritional info:
Calories: 242
Fat: 12.3 g
Cholesterol: 209 mg
Sodium: 579 mg
Carbohydrates: 8.9 g
Fibre: 2.8 g
Protein: 27.4 g

Mac And Cheese With Cauliflower

Mac and cheese is a pretty irreplaceable dish, but you can make a mean low carb version by swapping the pasta for cauliflower. This is a great recipe to have up your sleeve and it stands a good chance of being popular with kids as well as adults. If you find you really miss the pasta, you could make a compromise with half pasta and half cauliflower florets – but with this recipe, you may not need to!

Serves: 8

You will need:

- ½ teaspoon of butter
- 2 tablespoons of olive oil
- 170 g / 6 oz cream cheese
- 450 g / 4 cups cheddar cheese
- 450 g / 2 cups of mozzarella cheese
- 240 ml / 1 cup double cream / heavy cream
- Pinch of black pepper
- Pinch of salt
- 2 medium cauliflowers

Method:

1 Preheat your oven to 190 degrees C / 375 degrees F and use the butter to grease a large baking dish.

2 Wash your cauliflowers and chop them into florets.

3 Add the florets to a large bowl and toss them with the oil and a little salt.

4 Spread the cauliflower onto 2 baking sheets and put it in the oven to roast until tender (about 40 minutes).

5 Grate the cheddar and mozzarella cheeses.

6 In a large pan, heat the cream over a medium heat. Simmer gently and then lower the heat and stir in the cheeses, including the cream cheese. Keep stirring gently until they have fully melted.

7 Remove from the heat and season and then fold in the roasted cauliflower.

8 Tip the mixture into your baking dish and if you wish to add any toppings to your mac and cheese (e.g. extra cheese, dried herbs, etc.), do so.

9 Put back in the oven and bake for 15 minutes, until golden, and then serve hot.

Nutritional info:

Calories: 312

Fat: 22.1 g

Cholesterol: 60 mg

Sodium: 521 mg

Carbohydrates: 10 g

Fibre: 3.6 g

Protein: 20.5 g

Steak And Veggie Roast

If you're prepared to consume slightly more carbs at dinner than for your other meals, you'll love this sheet pan of steak and vegetables, and it makes a great luxury dinner that feels like a treat without going super heavy on the carbs. If you want to reduce the carbohydrate content, swap the potatoes for something like Brussels sprouts or green beans, and you'll still have a tasty recipe.

Serves: 6

You will need:

- 900 g / 2 pounds of inch thick top sirloin steak
- 3 cloves of garlic
- 900 g / 2 lb red potatoes
- 2 tablespoons of olive oil
- 450 g / 16 oz broccoli florets
- 1 teaspoon of thyme
- Pinch of salt
- Pinch of pepper

Method:

1   Preheat your oven to its top setting and oil a baking sheet.

2   Bring a large pot of water to the boil and wash and chop your potatoes. Boil them for about 12 minutes until they are starting to turn tender.

3   Wash and chop your broccoli.

4   Drain the potatoes and place them on the baking sheet, along with the broccoli florets.

5   Peel and slice your garlic and scatter it among the potatoes and broccoli, along with the thyme and olive oil. Season and gently stir to combine all the ingredients.

6   Pat your steaks to dry and slice them, and then scatter them among the vegetables in a single layer.

7   Place in the oven to broil, and turn the steak after 5 minutes. Continue to cook until the steak is brown and the vegetables are fully cooked. Make sure the steak has reached a minimum temperature of 49 degrees C / 120 degrees F for rare steak.

Nutritional info:

Calories: 455

Fat: 14.6 g

Cholesterol: 135 mg

Sodium: 161 mg

Carbohydrates: 29.7 g

Fibre: 4.6 g

Protein: 51 g

Scallops And Tomatoes In Butter

If you're feeling fancy, you'll love this scallop and tomato dish, which uses butter and capers to make a rich, salty sauce that brings out the full flavour of the scallops. You might want to make this with a low carb side such as cauliflower rice to bulk it out, but it's delicious as it is, too.

Serves: 4

You will need:

- 1 tablespoon of extra-virgin olive oil
- 400 g / 2 cups of cherry tomatoes
- 120 ml / ½ cup of dry white wine
- ¼ teaspoon of black pepper
- 2 tablespoons of capers
- 3 tablespoons of butter
- 450 g / 1 lb of dry sea scallops (remove the muscle)

- 10 g fresh parsley

Method:

1 Heat the oil in a large skillet over a medium heat. Pat your scallops dry and add them to the pan, cooking for a couple of minutes. Flip them over and cook them for another 2-3 minutes until they are golden. Put them in a bowl with a lid and set them aside.

2 Wash your cherry tomatoes and add them to the pan, gently cooking them until they start to turn brown and burst open.

3 Rinse your capers and add them to the pan, followed by the wine. Cook until the mixture has reduced by half, which should take a couple of minutes.

4 Take the pan off the heat, add the pepper, and then stir in the butter.

5 Serve the scallops with the sauce drizzled across the top and a garnishing of chopped parsley.

Nutritional info:

Calories: 249
Fat: 13.2 g
Cholesterol: 60 mg
Sodium: 379 mg
Carbohydrates: 7.4 g
Fibre: 1.3 g
Protein: 20.1 g

Butternut Squash Noodles With Smoked Salmon

If you're craving pasta, you can make amazing butternut squash noodles that are satisfyingly long and pasta-like. You can mix almost anything with these that you would usually have with spaghetti, including tomato sauce, but try them with some strips of smoked salmon for a really delicious and simple dinner.

Serves: 4

You will need:

- 2 tablespoons of extra-virgin olive oil
- 60 g / 2 oz of smoked salmon
- 40 g / 1 ½ oz of Parmesan
- 1 pinch of red pepper flakes
- 1 pinch of salt
- 1 pinch of pepper

- 450 g / 16 oz of butternut squash

Method:

1 Preheat your oven to 220 degrees C / 425 degrees F.

2 Peel your butternut squash and use a spiraliser to cut the flesh into long, thin strips like spaghetti.

3 Put the noodles on a large baking sheet and toss them with the red pepper flakes, olive oil, salt, and pepper. Place them in the oven and roast for 10 minutes.

4 Take the noodles out and stir them to check they are tender and hot.

5 Tear your salmon into strips and stir it through the noodles, and then serve with grated Parmesan. You can add other herbs, spices, or toppings if you like.

Nutritional info:

Calories: 161
Fat: 9.9 g
Cholesterol: 11 mg
Sodium: 436 mg
Carbohydrates: 13.7 g
Fibre: 2.3 g
Protein: 7.1 g

Buttery Garlic Meatballs With Courgette / Zucchini Noodles

You can enjoy your very own low carb version of spaghetti and meatballs using this great recipe – it swaps the meatballs for chicken balls to ensure the meat is lean, and the spaghetti for "zoodles." Zoodles are zucchini (courgette) noodles and they may well become a staple of your low carb diet, because you can eat them with anything you fancy!

Serves: 4

You will need:

- 1 egg
- 4 tablespoons of butter
- 450 g / 1 lb of ground chicken
- 5 cloves of garlic
- 40 g / 1 ½ oz Parmesan
- 2 tablespoons of extra-virgin olive oil
- ¼ teaspoon of red pepper flakes
- 1 tablespoon of lemon juice
- 2 tablespoons of parsley
- 450 g / 1 lb courgette / zucchini
- Pinch of salt
- Pinch of pepper

Method:

1 Get out a large mixing bowl and add the ground chicken. Peel and mince 2 cloves of garlic and stir them in, along with the grated Parmesan, red pepper flakes, egg, and chopped parsley. Add salt and pepper, and then form into meatballs.

2 Place a large skillet over a medium heat and warm the oil. When it starts to shimmer, add the meatballs and cook them until they are golden on all sides. They will take about 10 minutes to cook through. Check that they have reached at least 73 degrees C / 165 degrees F inside. When they have, place them on some paper towels to drain.

3 Melt the butter into the oil in the skillet and then peel and mince the remaining garlic. Add it to the butter and cook it for 1 minute.

4 Wash and spiralise your courgette / zucchini and toss it into the garlic butter, stirring to combine. Add the lemon juice and allow to cook for 2 minutes.

5 Add the meatballs back to the skillet and stir. Cook until everything is hot through and then serve with the option of additional Parmesan or cheddar cheese.

Nutritional info:

Calories: 453

Fat: 30.6 g

Cholesterol: 180 mg

Sodium: 346 mg

Carbohydrates: 5.8 g

Fibre: 1.5 g

Protein: 39.4 g

14 Day Diet Plan

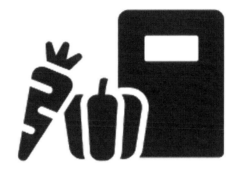

Day 1

Breakfast: Crustless Quiche

Let's start day one off with a satisfying, delicious breakfast that you can make in under an hour. The great thing about this quiche is that you can store it in the fridge and either eat it cold or heat it up very quickly in the microwave, so it makes a great breakfast option for days when you are too busy to deal with cooking in the morning.

Serves: 6

You will need:

- 8 large eggs
- 22 g / 0.7 oz of grated Parmesan
- 1 tablespoon of butter
- 225 g / 8 oz cremini mushrooms
- ½ onion
- 60 g / 2 cups of spinach
- 60 ml / ¼ cup of milk
- 15 g / ¼ cup of sun-dried tomatoes in oil
- Pinch of salt
- Pinch of pepper

Method:

1 Preheat your oven to 190 degrees C / 375 degrees F.

2 Wash your mushrooms and slice them thinly.

3 Place a skillet over a medium heat, add butter, and allow it to melt. Next, add the mushrooms and cook them for about 6 minutes, until they are golden and beginning to turn soft.

4 Peel and slice your onion and add it to the pan, and cook for 1 minute.

5 Wash the spinach and add it to the pan, and cook until wilted. Season the ingredients and take the pan off the heat.

6 Take out a large mixing bowl and whisk together the grated Parmesan, eggs, and milk. Slice your sun-dried tomatoes into fine strips and add them to the mixture.

7 Fold the mushrooms into the egg mixture and then pour the entire mix into a dish and bake until the eggs have set. This should take about 20 minutes, and the eggs should form a light crust on the outside of the quiche.

8 Stand the dish on the side and allow it cool for a few minutes, and then slice and serve hot, or eat cold.

Nutritional info:

Calories: 156

Fat: 10.4 g

Cholesterol: 256 mg

Sodium: 195 mg

Carbohydrates: 5 g

Fibre: 0.9 g

Protein: 11.5 g

Lunch: Aubergine / Eggplant Pizza (See page 44)

Dinner: Mac And Cheese With Cauliflower (See page 55)

DAY 2

Breakfast: Cream Cheese Pancakes (See page 20)

Lunch: Courgette / Zucchini Ragu (See page 41)

Dinner: Salmon, Potato, And Leek Bake

This delicious recipe is wonderfully filling, making it a perfect way to end the day. If you want to reduce the carbs in it further, use fewer potatoes, but it should still be low enough to be suitable for most low carb diets, especially if you keep your other meals low. This is a great way to get some healthy fish into your diet and it makes a delightful dinner for two.

Serves: 2

You will need:

- 2 tablespoons of olive oil
- 1 clove of garlic
- 2 salmon fillets
- 70 ml / 4 tablespoons of double cream / heavy cream
- 1 leek
- 1 tablespoon of chives

- 1 tablespoon of capers
- 50 g / 1 ½ oz of rocket / arugula
- 250 g / 8.8 oz of baby potatoes
- 75 ml / 1/3 of a cup of hot water

Method:

1. Preheat your oven to 200 degrees C / 390 degrees F.

2. Wash your potatoes and bring a pan of water to the boil while you cut them into thick slices. Add the slices to the pan and boil for about 8 minutes.

3. Drain the potatoes and leave them to dry for a few minutes, and then tip them into a baking dish and toss them with a tablespoon of olive oil and some seasoning.

4. Put the potatoes in the oven for 10 minutes and then take them out and toss them again, and put them back for another 10 minutes.

5. While the potatoes are cooking, add the remaining tablespoon of olive oil to a large skillet. Wash the leek and slice it into thin strips, and then fry it for several minutes until it starts to soften.

6. Crush your garlic and stir it in with the leek, and then add the capers, the cream, and the hot water. Bring it to a gentle boil, making sure it doesn't stick, and stir in some chopped chives.

7. Put your grill on a high heat. Take the potatoes out of the oven and pour your leeks and cream over them, stirring gently to combine. Place the salmon fillets on top and then grill for around 8 minutes, until the salmon reaches an internal temperature of at least 60 degrees C / 145 degrees F, and the flesh is flaky and tender.

8 Top with extra chives and capers, and serve with the washed rocket / arugula.

Nutritional info:

Calories: 588
Fat: 38.6 g
Cholesterol: 127 mg
Sodium: 248 mg
Carbohydrates: 24.5 g
Fibre: 4.5 g
Protein: 40 g

Day 3

Breakfast: Toasted Nuts And Cottage Cheese Bowl (See page 27)

Lunch: Mediterranean Mackerel Salad (See page 47)

Dinner: Garlicky Spaghetti Squash

Many people find that they miss pasta dishes more than any other meal, and if you're used to throwing together a quick pasta for dinner, you might be particularly struggling with the evening meal. Spaghetti is not low in carbs, but you can use a spaghetti squash to replicate the texture beautifully – and this garlicky dinner is a perfect option for enjoying a pasta-like meal without the carbs.

Serves: 2

You will need:

- 1 tablespoon of olive oil
- 3 cloves of garlic
- 450 g / 1 lb of spaghetti squash
- 45 g / ½ cup of Parmesan
- 2 tablespoons of fresh parsley

- 1 tablespoon of butter
- 240 ml / 1 cup of chicken stock
- 5 tablespoons of sour cream
- Pinch of salt
- Pinch of pepper

Method:

1 Wash your spaghetti squash and cut off the ends. Slice it lengthwise into 2 pieces, and then scrape the seeds out of the centre.

2 Place it in a microwave-safe dish with the inside of the vegetable facing down, and add about an inch of water. Microwave it for about 6 minutes, and then allow it to rest for a minute. Microwave it for another 6 minutes and check whether it is tender. If not, give it a longer. If it is, use a fork to separate out the strands and put them into a clean bowl.

3 Place a large pan over a medium heat and add the butter and olive oil. Mince the garlic and cook for 1 minute, and then add the chicken stock and bring to a boil.

4 Add the strands of spaghetti squash and cook for 2 minutes. Next, remove the saucepan from the heat and stir in the Parmesan. Add the sour cream, and then cook on a low heat for 2 more minutes, stirring well so that it doesn't stick or burn.

5 Garnish with freshly chopped parsley and some additional Parmesan, plus salt and pepper. Serve hot.

Nutritional info:

Calories: 330
Fat: 25.5 g
Cholesterol: 45 mg
Sodium: 772 mg
Carbohydrates: 19.8 g
Fibre: 0.2 g
Protein: 10.4 g

Day 4

Breakfast: Cream Cheese Pancakes (See page 20)

Lunch: Chicken With Pesto Veggies

If you need a simple, tasty lunch that you can take to work with you or eat from home, chicken with pesto veggies is a great option that will leave you feeling full and get some of those crucial 5 a day into your diet. You can alter the vegetables if you like, but remember to choose low carb options to keep the overall carbohydrate count down.

> Serves: 4

You will need:

- 115 g / ½ cup of pesto
- 455 g / 1 lb of green beans
- 2 tablespoons of olive oil
- 400 g / 2 cups of cherry tomatoes
- 4 boneless, skinless chicken thighs
- Pinch of salt
- Pinch of pepper

Method:

1   Heat the oil in a large skillet and add the chicken thighs, plus seasoning. Cook until the chicken is fully done and has reached an internal temperature of 75 degrees C / 165 degrees F.

2   Set the chicken aside to cool and then slice it into thin strips.

3   Add the green beans to the pan and cook until they turn tender, and then toss the chicken back in too. Stir in the pesto.

4   Wash and halve your cherry tomatoes and add these to the pan. Stir well so the ingredients are fully mixed and then turn off the heat and serve the meal, or chill in the fridge.

Nutritional info:

Calories: 634

Fat: 25.4 g

Cholesterol: 380 mg

Sodium: 451 mg

Carbohydrates: 12.1 g

Fibre: 5.1 g

Protein: 91 g

Dinner: Steak And Veggie Roast (See page 58)

Day 5

Breakfast: Blueberry Muffins

Sometimes, you want a breakfast that tastes good and feels like comfort food, but you don't want to ruin all your hard work so far. If you are starting to struggle by the time day 5 rolls around, you might want to kick-start the day with a warm, comforting muffin – and these blueberry muffins will be fine on the carb count for most low carb diets. They are easy to make and can be stored in an airtight container or frozen until you want them.

Serves: 12

You will need:

- 3 eggs
- 1 tablespoon of coconut flour
- 1 teaspoon of baking powder
- 2 tablespoons of coconut oil
- 1 tablespoon of vanilla extract
- 1 teaspoon of lemon zest
- 2 tablespoons of lemon juice
- 170 g / 1 ½ cups of almond flour
- 250 g / ¾ cup of honey
- ½ teaspoon of salt
- 140 g / ¾ cup of blueberries

Method:

1 Preheat the oven to 175 degrees C / 350 degrees F.

2 Take out a large mixing bowl and sift together the coconut flour, almond flour, salt, and baking powder.

3 In a second bowl, whisk together the honey, vanilla extract, coconut oil (melted), lemon juice, lemon zest, and eggs.

4 Tip a little of the honey and egg mixture into the flour mixture and stir until fully combined. Keep gradually adding the honey and eggs and mixing thoroughly until you have a smooth, runny batter.

5 Wash the blueberries and fold them into the mixture, and then grease your muffin trays and pour some mixture into each hole.

6 Bake for about 20 minutes and then use a toothpick to check whether they are cooked through. Serve warm or enjoy cold.

Nutritional info:

Calories: 196

Fat: 10.1 g

Cholesterol: 41 mg

Sodium: 100 mg

Carbohydrates: 22.7 g

Fibre: 2 g

Protein: 4.6 g

Lunch: Aubergine / Eggplant Pizza (See page 44)

Dinner: Scallops And Tomatoes In Butter (See page 61)

Day 6

Breakfast: Banana Bread (See page 22)

Lunch: Simple Mushrooms And Kale

If you want a lunch that is really low in carbs but still packed with goodness and nutrients, this mushroom and kale mix is perfect. You can make it in under half an hour using just one pan, and it's a delicious way to break up the day.

Serves: 4

You will need:

- 4 eggs
- 1 tablespoon of olive oil
- 2 cloves of garlic
- 250 g / 8.8 oz mushrooms
- 160 g / 5.6 oz kale

Method:

1 Wash your mushrooms and slice them into thick chunks. Peel the garlic cloves and crush them.

2 Heat the olive oil in a large skillet over a medium heat and then fry the garlic gently for 1 minute. Add the mushrooms to the pan and cook until soft.

3 Wash the kale and shake it dry, and then start adding it to the pan. Depending on the size of the pan, you may need to add it a little at a time, but be aware that it will cook down a lot. Allow it to wilt fully and then add seasoning if you choose.

4 One at a time, crack the eggs carefully into the pan, spacing them out among the other ingredients. You may want to make some hollows using a wooden spoon first.

5 Cook until the eggs are firm and to your liking.

Nutritional info:

Calories: 128

Fat: 8.1 g

Cholesterol: 164 mg

Sodium: 83 mg

Carbohydrates: 7.1 g

Fibre: 1.3 g

Protein: 8.8 g

Dinner: Buttery Garlic Meatballs With Courgette / Zucchini Noodles (See page 66)

DAY 7

Breakfast: Shakshuka (See page 31)

Lunch: Lemony Chicken And Avocado Salad

If you're a salad fan, this light, fresh recipe is the one for you – and it's very low on carbs. You can make this in batches and take it to work with you, or enjoy it at home. This is an ideal way to keep your carb count low in the middle of the day without trying to skip meals or missing out on a tasty lunch.

Serves: 6

You will need:

- 2 medium avocados
- 3 teaspoons of mayonnaise
- 420 g / 3 cups of cooked chicken
- 40 g / ¼ cup of spring onion / green onion
- 2 teaspoons of chopped coriander / cilantro
- 3 teaspoons of lemon juice
- Pinch of salt

Method:

1. Cut your cooked chicken into large chunks and then dice the avocados and add both ingredients to a large mixing bowl with 1 teaspoon of lemon juice and a little salt.

2. Peel and dice your spring onion / green onion and chop the coriander / cilantro.

3. Mix the remaining lemon juice with the mayonnaise and taste. Adjust the flavour if necessary.

4. Add the onions and dressing to the chicken and avocado and toss the mixture thoroughly until the chicken and avocado are coated. Gently stir in the coriander / cilantro.

5. Chill and then serve cold.

Nutritional info:

Calories: 254

Fat: 16.1 g

Cholesterol: 55 mg

Sodium: 94 mg

Carbohydrates: 6.8 g

Fibre: 4.7 g

Protein: 21.7 g

Dinner: Garlic-Infused Shrimp And Broccoli (See page 52)

DAY 8

Breakfast: Baked Egg Avocados (See page 25)

Lunch: Mediterranean Mackerel Salad (See page 47)

Dinner: Amazing Salmon Burgers

Not all fish meals need to be cooked in sauces or made to look fancy – you can make some really simple salmon burgers to enjoy as part of your low carb diet. These are great for freezing and then whipping up into a fast, healthy dinner. You can serve them with a side salad or with a vegetable such as peas or green beans. Avoid bread or rice.

Serves: 4

You will need:

- 1 tablespoon of Thai red curry paste
- 1 teaspoon of soy sauce
- 30 g / 1 oz of coriander / cilantro
- 1 teaspoon of vegetable oil

- 550 g / 1 lb 4 oz of salmon fillets (skinless, boneless)
- 1 thumb of ginger (approx. 25 g / 0.8 oz)
- 4 lemon wedges

Method:

1 If you have a food processor, use it to chop and mix the salmon, soy sauce, ginger, Thai red curry paste and coriander / cilantro. If you don't have a food processor, chop the salmon by hand and mix it thoroughly with the grated ginger, chopped coriander / cilantro, soy sauce, and Thai red curry paste. You should get a thick mixture.

2 Tip this onto a clean surface and shape it into four burgers.

3 Add oil to a non-stick skillet and warm over a medium heat, and then fry the burgers for around 5 minutes. Flip them and fry for another 5 minutes, until they are crispy and hot through.

4 Serve piping hot or space out to cool and freeze.

Nutritional info:

Calories: 84

Fat: 4.7 g

Cholesterol: 6 mg

Sodium: 477 mg

Carbohydrates: 7 g

Fibre: 1.2 g

Protein: 3.6 g

DAY 9

Breakfast: Green Eggs

If you've got eggs and spinach, it will only take you about 15 minutes to whip up this delicious baked eggs recipe, and it's a great way to start your day with as few carbs as possible. Eggs make a nice, filling meal, and with some spinach in there too, you've got a fantastic breakfast with plenty of iron and nutrients.

Serves: 2

You will need:

- 4 eggs
- 1 tablespoon of cheddar cheese (or another cheese of your choice)
- 4 tablespoons of pesto
- 100 g / 3 ½ oz of baby spinach
- 100 ml / 3 tablespoons of double cream / heavy cream

Method:

1. Preheat your oven to 200 degrees C / 390 degrees F.

2. Wash and chop your baby spinach into rough chunks, and then use a large bowl to mix it with the pesto and cream.

3. Tip the mixture into 2 ovenproof dishes and sprinkle grated cheese across the top.

4. Use a wooden spoon to make 2 shallow dents in the ingredients in both dishes, and add an egg to each of these hollows.

5. Bake for up to 12 minutes, until the eggs are set. The yolks should still be runny. If you would rather have them firm, add a few more minutes to your cooking time.

Nutritional info:

Calories: 462

Fat: 41.9 g

Cholesterol: 408 mg

Sodium: 394 mg

Carbohydrates: 6 g

Fibre: 1.6 g

Protein: 17.4 g

Lunch: Chicken Caesar Salad (See page 38)

Dinner: Steak And Veggie Roast (See page 58)

Day 10

Breakfast: Shakshuka (See page 31)

Lunch: Ham And Broccoli Salad

You can make this tasty salad in advance and store it in the fridge to ensure you've always got a quick and easy lunch to hand. If you aren't fond of ham, feel free to swap this for another lean meat, or adjust the quantities of cauliflower and broccoli to suit your tastes. This salad needs to be served with a dressing, so pick your favourite or whip up your own with oil and vinegar, and enjoy!

Serves: 4

You will need:

- ½ head of cauliflower
- 250 g / 9 oz broccoli
- 225 g / 8 oz mozzarella cubes
- 20 g / 0.7 oz Parmesan
- 200 g / 1 cup of cherry tomatoes
- 130 g / 1 cup of ham
- 90 g / ½ cup of olives

Method:

1   Thoroughly wash your broccoli and cauliflower, and chop both into small florets.

2   Halve the cherry tomatoes and olives, and cut the mozzarella into cubes.

3   Get a large salad bowl and mix together all of the ingredients, and then toss them in dressing to coat them.

Nutritional info:

Calories: 289
Fat: 16.1 g
Cholesterol: 53 mg
Sodium: 1006 mg
Carbohydrates: 12.3 g
Fibre: 4 g
Protein: 26.2 g

Dinner: Scallops And Tomatoes In Butter (See page 61)

Breakfast: Cauliflower Toast

For those wanting a simple breakfast, cauliflower toast is a nice, easy option. With a little bit of cheese and no bread anywhere in sight, this will get you off to a great start for the day, although it takes a little longer to make than some of the other breakfast options in this book.

Serves: 5

You will need:

- 1 large egg
- 1 teaspoon of garlic powder (or a clove of garlic)
- 1 medium cauliflower
- 60 g / ½ cup of cheese
- Pinch of salt
- Pinch of pepper

Method:

1 Preheat your oven to 220 degrees C / 425 degrees F and line a baking tray with some greaseproof paper / parchment paper.

2 Use a grater to grate your cauliflower and tip it into a microwave-safe bowl. Microwave it on high for 8 minutes and then drain it on a clean towel until dry.

3 Tip the cauliflower back into the bowl and grate in the cheese. Next, add your egg and garlic powder, and season. Mix thoroughly.

4 Lift portions of the cauliflower onto your baking sheet and shape it into bread-like shapes. Put it into the oven and bake for about 20 minutes, until it is lightly golden. Gently transfer it to a plate and add any savoury toppings that take your fancy.

Nutritional info:

Calories: 49
Fat: 1.8 g
Cholesterol: 40 mg
Sodium: 130 mg
Carbohydrates: 3.5 g
Fibre: 1.4 g
Protein: 5.2 g

Lunch: Cheesy Mushrooms (See page 36)

Dinner: Garlic-Infused Shrimp And Broccoli (See page 52)

DAY 12

Breakfast: Baked Egg Avocados (See page 25)

Lunch: Smoked Salmon, Rocket / Arugula, And Avocado Salad

This can also stand in as a great breakfast recipe, but most people enjoy eating it for lunch. It makes a wonderfully light meal that is perfect for hot days. It's also beautifully simple and can be tossed together with very little time and effort. Again, you can choose whatever dressing you like for this salad, or just squeeze a dash of lemon juice across it to complement the fish.

Serves: 1

You will need:

- ½ avocado
- 1 tablespoon sesame seeds
- ¼ cucumber
- 60 g / 2 oz rocket / arugula
- 100 g / 3 oz smoked salmon
- ½ teaspoon of lemon juice

Method:

1 Place a pan on the stove and add the sesame seeds but no oil. Lightly toast the seeds for a couple of minutes until they have turned gently brown.

2 Wash and dry the rocket / arugula and set it to one side.

3 Wash and slice your cucumber into thin slices.

4 Add your rocket leaves and cucumber to a bowl and tear the smoked salmon into pieces and toss these in too.

5 Slice your avocado and squeeze a little lemon juice over it to prevent it from browning. Stir it into the rest of the ingredients, scatter a handful of sesame seeds over the top, and add a dressing if you want to. Leave the dressing off the salad and add it to the individual portions to help the salad stay fresh.

Nutritional info:

Calories: 400
Fat: 28.9 g
Cholesterol: 24 mg
Sodium: 2025 mg
Carbohydrates: 15.7 g
Fibre: 9.1 g
Protein: 23.9 g

Dinner: Butternut Squash Noodles With Smoked Salmon (See page 64)

Day 13

Breakfast: Banana Bread (See page 22)

Lunch: Courgette / Zucchini Ragu (See page 41)

Dinner: Lemony Garlic Salmon Bake

Salmon is a great staple ingredient for your low carb meals, and you can make this delicious lemon and salmon dish with asparagus spears in under half an hour. You can adjust the vegetables that are on offer if you like, but make sure you choose low carb options. If you want a more luxurious meal, consider adding a dollop of plain Greek yoghurt / yogurt to serve with the salmon.

Serves: 6

You will need:

- Cooking spray
- 1 lemon
- 45 g / 1/3 cup of peas
- 170 g / 6 oz salmon fillets
- 3 cloves of garlic
- 2 tablespoons of parsley
- 1 teaspoon of salt
- ½ teaspoon of pepper
- 4 bunches of asparagus
- 80 ml / 1/3 cup of lemon juice

Method:

1 Heat your oven to 230 degrees C / 450 degrees F and line a baking sheet with foil.

2 Put your salmon on the sheet and mince your garlic. Rub the garlic and chopped parsley into the salmon thoroughly, and then pour lemon juice across the top.

3 Wash your asparagus and cut off the woody ends, and then arrange this around the salmon. Spread the peas onto the baking sheet too.

4 Lightly spray or brush the ingredients with olive oil and add a little salt and pepper.

5 Slice your lemon and place the slices on the ingredients.

6 Grill the salmon for about 8-10 minutes and then check that it is cooked through. Do not let it burn, since the oven will be very hot.

Nutritional info:

Calories: 73

Fat: 2.2 g

Cholesterol: 13 mg

Sodium: 406 mg

Carbohydrates: 6.8 g

Fibre: 2.9 g

Protein: 8.4 g

DAY 14

Breakfast: Toasted Nuts And Cottage Cheese Bowl (See page 27)

Lunch: Chicken Caesar Salad (See page 38)

Dinner: Shrimp And Courgette / Zucchini Noodles

We've already covered these alternative noodles, but they are ideal for this recipe with shrimps, so don't under-utilize them – they are one of the quickest ways to throw together a meal when you're not in the mood to cook, but they also look amazing. All you need is a spiraliser and you've got magazine-worthy noodles to enjoy, and they work beautifully with the shrimps!

Serves: 4

You will need:

- 450 g / 1 lb of shrimps, peeled and deveined
- 2 tablespoons of white wine
- ½ onion
- 2 tablespoons of butter
- 2 cloves of garlic
- 3 tablespoons of olive oil
- 55 g / 2 oz of Parmesan

- 2 tablespoons of fresh parsley
- 200 g / 1 cup of cherry tomatoes
- ½ teaspoon of black pepper
- 2 tablespoons of chicken stock (unsalted)
- 115 g / 6 cups of zucchini

Method:

1. Add 1 tablespoon of oil and 1 tablespoon of butter to a large skillet and place it over a medium heat so that the butter melts. Meanwhile, peel and slice your onion, and then add this to the pan.

2. Cook the onion until it has softened and then peel and mince the garlic and add this to the pan. Cook for 1 minute.

3. Add the chicken stock and wine, and allow to cook for about 2 minutes until it reduces.

4. Clean, peel, and devein the shrimps, and then add them to the pan and season with black pepper.

5. Cook for about 2 minutes and then turn and cook for another 1-2 minutes, until the shrimp are cooked through.

6. Put the shrimps on a plate and set them aside, leaving the other ingredients in the skillet.

7   Wash and halve your cherry tomatoes and toss them into the sauce, along with the rest of your oil. Cook for about 1 minute, until tomatoes are soft.

8   Wash and spiralise your courgettes / zucchinis and add them to the skillet, tossing all the ingredients to combine them.

9   Put the shrimps back in and cook for 1-2 minutes, so everything is hot. Remove the pan from the heat and add half of the Parmesan, and then serve with chopped parsley and the remaining Parmesan.

Nutritional info:

Calories: 372

Fat: 21.6 g

Cholesterol: 264 mg

Sodium: 491 mg

Carbohydrates: 12.1 g

Fibre: 2.9 g

Protein: 33.2 g

Conclusion

Hopefully, you now have a good range of recipes to try out and enjoy! Reducing your carbohydrates is certainly one of the best ways to improve your health, make yourself feel better, and lower your weight, but it can be a challenge if you don't have some good recipes on standby. It's so easy to fall back on bread, pasta, oats, rice, and other carbohydrate-laden foods, and while these are fine in small quantities, you need to avoid them where possible!

In today's society, we depend far too much on these easy foods, and it can be really difficult to get away from them. Fortunately, you can take control in your kitchen and start making your meals with far fewer carbohydrates. Wherever possible, swap grains for vegetables and don't be afraid to experiment with different flavours.

Things like cauliflowers and broccoli are enormously versatile and can be used to make all sorts of substitute dishes – so give them a chance to shine in your meals. Remember to use herbs and spices to boost the flavours and make sure you can really enjoy your food.

EXCLUSIVE BONUS

40 Weight Loss Recipes

&

14 Days Meal Plan

Scan the QR-Code and receive
the FREE download:

Disclaimer

This book contains opinions and ideas of the author and is meant to teach the reader informative and helpful knowledge while due care should be taken by the user in the application of the information provided. The instructions and strategies are possibly not right for every reader and there is no guarantee that they work for everyone. Using this book and implementing the information/recipes therein contained is explicitly your own responsibility and risk. This work with all its contents, does not guarantee correctness, completion, quality or correctness of the provided information. Misinformation or misprints cannot be completely eliminated.

-

Printed in Great Britain
by Amazon